MW01275603

Lunch With Quinn

The story of one child's diagnosis and management of Celiac Disease

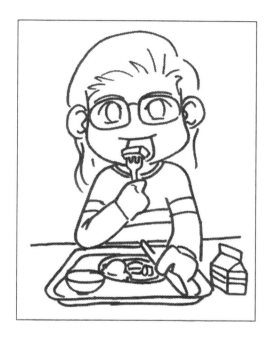

Written by
Angela Porter

Illustrations by
Jae Hong Choi

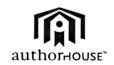

authorHOUSE™

1663 LIBERTY DRIVE, SUITE 200
BLOOMINGTON, INDIANA 47403
(800) 839-8640
WWW.AUTHORHOUSE.COM

© *2006 Angela Porter Illustrations by Jae Hong Choi. All rights reserved.*

No part of this book may be reproduced, stored in a retrieval system, or transmitted by any means without the written permission of the author.

First published by AuthorHouse 4/12/2006

ISBN: 1-4259-0699-0 (sc)

Library of Congress Control Number: 2005910960

Printed in the United States of America
Bloomington, Indiana

This book is printed on acid-free paper.

Dedicated to
My daughter,
Quinnlyn Alise Morton,
my own little 'silly act' kid
who has brought me nothing but
love, happiness and pleasure.

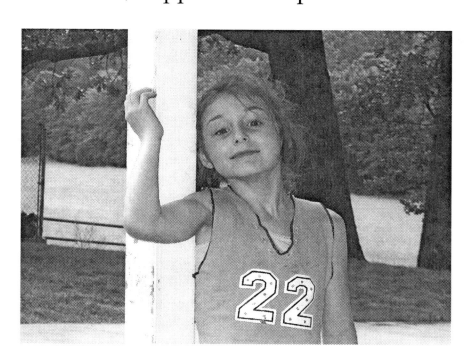

Special thanks to
Theresa Inman
for proofreading and correcting my
grammatical errors.

And to Nita Hatcher, food service
manager for Paris School District and all
of the cafeteria ladies at
Paris Elementary for always making
sure Quinn has a gluten free lunch at
school.

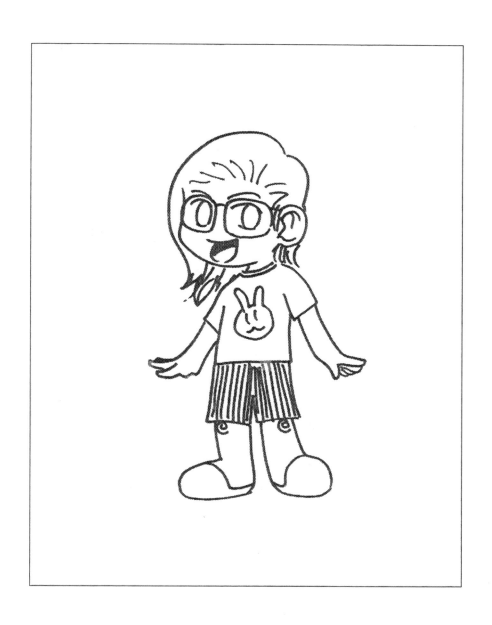

This is Quinn.
Quinn is five years old and in
kindergarten.

Quinn is a lot like most kindergartners.

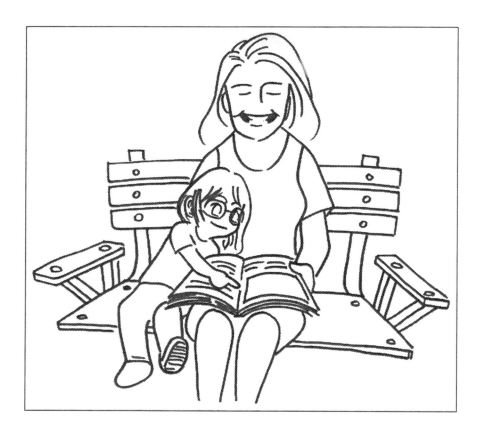

She likes to ride her bike, snuggle with her mom and read books.

And like a lot of kindergartners, Quinn does not like to clean her room, pick up her messes or go to bed.

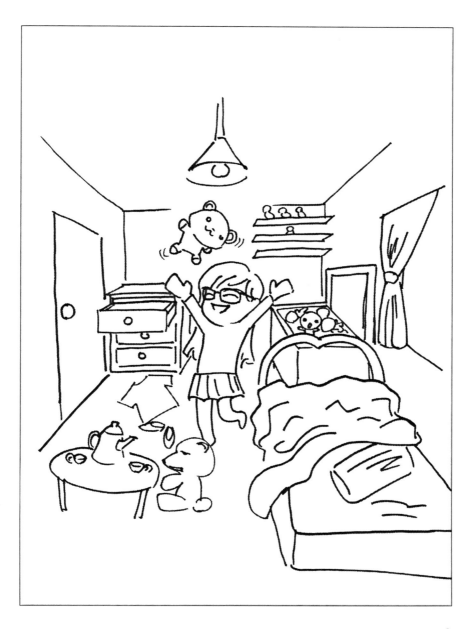

There is one big difference between Quinn and the rest of her class. Quinn is a Celiac kid (pronounced Silly Act).

Being a Celiac Kid does not mean Quinn acts silly, even though some times she does.

Being Celiac means that Quinn can not eat gluten. Gluten is something found in wheat, rye, barley and oat plants.

These plants are used to make flour that is used in lots of foods.

Most people can eat gluten without any problem. But Celiac Kids, like Quinn, will have tummy trouble if they eat any gluten.

So, when Quinn eats, she can not eat foods that have wheat, rye, barley or oats in them.

Some of these foods are,

bread   cereal   pizza

cookies   macaroni and   cake
                 cheese

biscuits and gravy,
which was Quinn's favorite food.
She would eat it everyday if her mom
would let her.

Quinn eats lunch in the cafeteria at her school. The cafeteria serves lots of foods that contain gluten, so eating in the cafeteria was a problem for Quinn.

But Mrs. Nita, the dietary manager at Quinn's school, learned as much as she could about Celiac Disease and gluten. She makes sure that Quinn always has a gluten free lunch at school, even if what Quinn gets for lunch is different from what the other students get for lunch.

How did Quinn find out she has Celiac disease? Well, she had lots of tummy trouble. For one thing, her tummy hurt all the time.

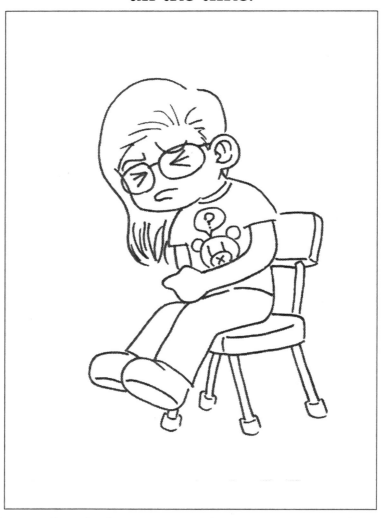

Everybody's tummy hurts some of the time, but Quinn's tummy hurt <u>all</u> the time.

Another thing that let Quinn know something was wrong with her tummy was she had to go to the bathroom to poop four or five times every day.

Most people only poop one or maybe two times a day, not five.

Also, Quinn would get sick to her tummy about once every week. She would wake up sick to her tummy in the middle of the night and throw up. Usually she would throw up all over the bed.

Then her Mommy would have to change the sheets on her bed.

One day Quinn's mommy took her to a special tummy doctor called a **Gastroenterologist**.

The doctor said she needed to look at Quinn's tummy so she could see what was wrong.

Quinn raised her shirt and showed the doctor her tummy. The doctor explained that she would have to look at the inside of Quinn's tummy.
She said she would have to do that at the hospital with a special camera.

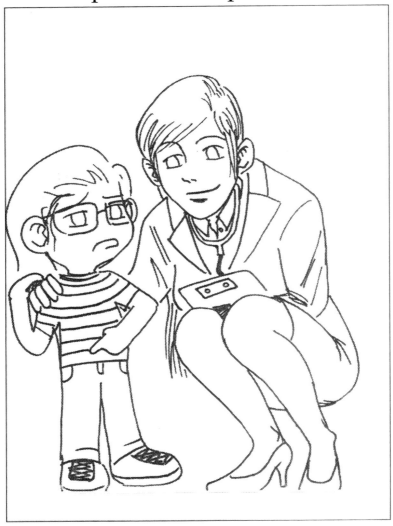

Early one morning, while it was still dark outside, Quinn, her mommy, and her Aunt Gee, whose real name is Jennifer but Quinn calls her Gee, went to the hospital.

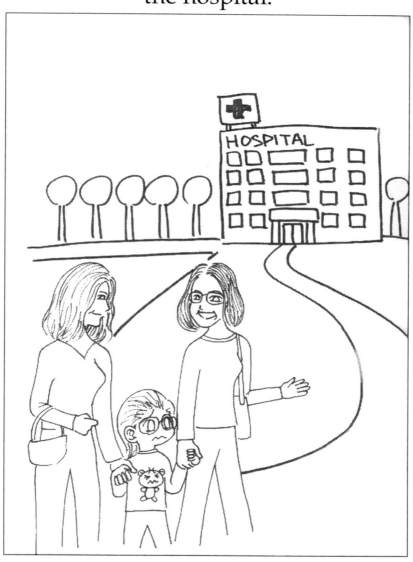

The nurses at the hospital helped Quinn put on a hospital gown. Then they gave her some medicine they called 'goofy juice' to help Quinn relax and go to sleep. Then a nurse took Quinn to a room where the doctor kept her special camera.

The doctor looked down Quinn's throat to her tummy and took some pictures. She also took some blood out of Quinn's arm while she was asleep.

When Quinn woke, up her mommy and Aunt Gee were with her. The doctor told them that she would call them when she found out from the blood and the pictures what was wrong with Quinn's tummy.

A few days later the doctor called. She said she knew what was wrong with Quinn's tummy.
Quinn and her mommy went to see the doctor. That's when they learned Quinn is a Celiac Kid.

The doctor explained that Celiac is a disease that if a person eats any gluten the gluten will hurt her intestines. The intestines are part of the body where food goes after it leaves the tummy. The intestines absorb vitamins and other nutrients the body needs to keep itself fed and healthy.

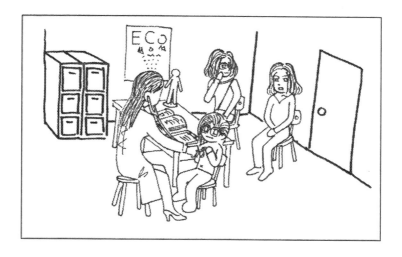

Quinn asked how she got celiac disease. Her doctor told her she was born with it. Celiac disease is not contagious, which means that Quinn's friends can not get it from her.

The doctor went on to explain that the lining of the intestines have little bumps called villi that absorb the vitamins and other nutrients. When a person with celiac eats any gluten the gluten "rubs off" the bumps. This keeps the person from absorbing what she needs and makes her tummy hurt. It also causes her to have to poop more often and sometimes throw up like Quinn would do.

The doctor told Quinn she could no longer eat foods with gluten or even foods that touch gluten.

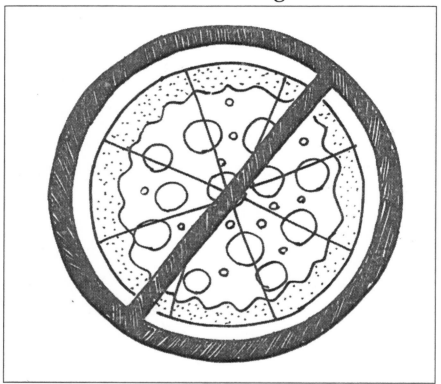

That means Quinn can not just pull the toppings off pizza. Because the toppings had touched the crust, they might have gotten some gluten on them that would make Quinn sick.

At first Quinn was upset because there were so many foods she could no longer eat. But the doctor said she had to stop eating those foods so her tummy would get better.

So, Quinn stopped eating foods with gluten. After a couple of weeks, Quinn stopped getting sick to her tummy at night. A week later she was only pooping one or two times a day.

But best of all, Quinn's tummy stopped
hurting all the time like it did before. If
Quinn happens to cheat or accidentally
eat something with gluten, her tummy
will hurt. So, Quinn does not cheat.

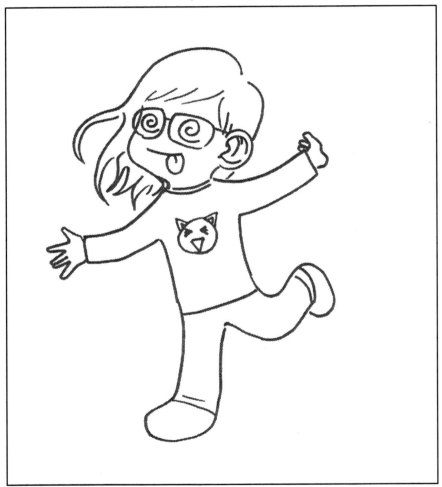

Quinn has learned that there are lots
Of good foods she can eat
that do not have gluten in them.

Some foods without gluten are

yogurt	grapes	potatoes
chicken	egg	corn
green beans	popcorn	bananas
apples	peanut butter	oranges

and rice, which is Quinn's new favorite
food.

Quinn's mom worried about what Quinn would eat at school, until she talked to Mrs. Nita and learned that she would take care of Quinn at lunch. Lots of days they serve food in the cafeteria that Quinn can not eat. So, on those days Quinn gets a different lunch from the rest of her class.

At first Quinn's friends did not understand why Quinn got a different lunch than they did. At first some of the kids would tease her because her lunch was different. After she explained about celiac disease and how some foods would hurt her tummy if she ate them, the kids stopped teasing her.

So, if you eat lunch with Quinn and she gets a different meal than you, now you know why.

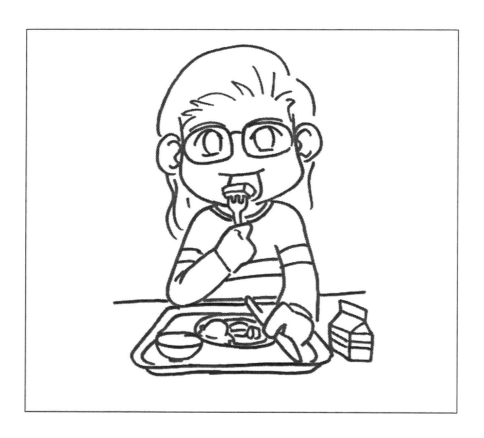

Facts about Celiac Disease

Celiac Disease is a condition that involves the small intestines. Those affected by Celiac disease have intolerance to the protein gluten that is found in wheat, rye, barley and oat grains. This intolerance causes destruction of the villi that absorb nutrients in foods. A person with Celiac Disease who eats gluten will be malnourished no matter how much food they eat because the nutrients are not getting into the body.

While there is no cure for Celiac Disease there is treatment. Treatment involves avoiding gluten. While this sounds easy enough, the truth is that gluten is 'hidden' in many common, everyday foods. Since even small amounts of gluten can cause problems for those with Celiac Disease, so labels must be read carefully to make sure products are gluten free. It is an absolute must for the Celiac and their family to understand that the gluten free diet must be strictly adhered to if the Celiac individual is to be healthy.

Author's Note

My daughter Quinn was our third child. Almost from the day she was born she would vomit much more frequently than my other children did. Many times I voiced concern to her Pediatrician who assured me that as long as she was growing she was fine. He even told me that I was a nervous, over-concerned mother. Not only was Quinn my third child but I am a pediatric nurse. Mothers know, have a sixth sense, when it comes to their children. I knew something was wrong. Quinn was breast fed until she was a year old so I knew the problem was not formula related. Unfortunately, our insurance dictated which group of Pediatricians I used so I was unable to change her doctor. As Quinn got older she continued to have bouts of vomiting in the night and her stools were more frequent and very full of fat. Fatty stools have a horrible smell and they tend to float.

When Quinn was about three I changed jobs and so did our insurance and Quinn's Pediatrician. Her new Pediatrician took more interest and greater care in Quinn's symptoms. By this time Quinn had also developed allergy symptoms, runny nose, dark circles under her eyes and congestion. Her physician thought the two may be related and treated the allergy symptoms. Quinn continued to vomit periodically at night and have frequent fatty stools.

When Quinn was five she had to see an ear, nose and throat (ENT) specialist for an unrelated problem. One look at her throat and the ENT asked if she vomited a lot. I told her she did. He said, "this needs to be checked out". I made another appointment with her Pediatrician and told her I wanted a referral for a pediatric Gastroenterologist (GI).

I can not explain the relief I had after the first visit with the GI doctor. My concerns were validated, it was not normal for a child to vomit like she did nor have the fatty stools. An appointment was made for an upper GI endoscopy, which involved outpatient surgery and allowed the doctor to see into Quinn's esophagus, stomach and small intestines. It also allowed for biopsies or small pieces of Quinn's esophagus, stomach and small intestines to be taken for further study. Blood was also drawn for analysis of Celiac Disease antibodies because once the doctor saw Quinn's small intestines she suspected the disease.

It is always hard to hear your child has a chronic illness, however, knowing something is wrong but not knowing what is even harder. A gluten free diet is not easy. But luckily there is a lot of information available on reading labels and foods both to avoid and that are 'safe'. I have contacted many well-known food companies to ask questions about specific products. So far I have had questions answered professionally and in some cases additional information has been sent to me in writing regarding gluten free foods the company produces.

Almost instantly we could see a change in Quinn, the vomiting stopped so did the fatty stools. The dark circles under her eyes disappeared. Before she was eating constantly, because she was malnourished and not getting the nutrients she needed because of the damage to her villi caused by the disease, she was starting to fall off the growth chart for her age. Now she eats regular meals and has gained some weight so that she is where she should be for her age and height.

Parents know when something is wrong with their child. As parents we must advocate or stand up for our children, as they can not speak for themselves. Quinn's prognosis is excellent, in part because her disease was caught and diet treatment began before further damage, irreparable damage could occur to her intestines. If you have a child and you suspect Celiac Disease or any other health problem I urge you to seek help and keep seeking it until your child gets the help they need. Remember…you are the expert when it comes to your child.

Angela Porter

About the author

Angela Porter is the mother of Quinn, a child with Celiac Disease. She has been with Quinn through vomiting, diarrhea, tummy aches and all physician and hospital visits. Angela is also a registered nurse with a Master's degree in nursing.

CPSIA information can be obtained
at www.ICGtesting.com
Printed in the USA
LVOW08s0022110417
530355LV00001B/60/P

9 781425 906993